MW00930196

ALL **WHAT TO EXPECT** WHEN YOU ARE **EXPECTING** MADE EASY (FROM MONTH 1 – 9)

A comprehensive guide to everything you need to know, from conception to birth and beyond. Also includes a week-by-week overview of your baby

And more

Jessie J Spear

Copyright© 2023**Jessie J Spear**

All rights reserved. No part or part of this book or publication may be reproduced, stored, or transferred in any form by electronic, mechanical, recording, or other retrieval system without written permission. of the publisher or author.

CONTENTS

CHAPTER ONE 9

THE STAGES OF PREGNANCY...........9

CHAPTER TWO....................18

NAVIGATING COMMON PREGNANCY SYMPTOMS AND DISCOMFORTS....18

CHAPTER THREE 28

THE EMOTIONAL ROLLER MOUNTAINS 28

CHAPTER FOUR....................46

NUTRITIONAL TIPS FOR HEALTHY PREGNANCY AND FETAL DEVELOPMENT 46

CHAPTER FIVE...................................**60**

STAYING ACTIVE WHILE PREGNANT: SAFE EXERCISE AND FITNESS ROUTINES 60

CHAPTER SIX **70**

PREPARING FOR LABOR AND CHILDBIRTH....................................70

CHAPTER SEVEN **81**

UNDERSTANDING PRENATAL SCREENINGS AND TESTS 81

CHAPTER EIGHT **90**

CREATE A BIRTH PLAN ADAPTED TO YOUR PREFERENCES AND NEEDS ...90

CHAPTER NINE............................**101**

DEALING WITH PREGNANCY-RELATED COMPLICATIONS AND HIGH-RISK SITUATIONS 101

CHAPTER TEN **111**

ROLE OF PARTNERS 111

CHAPTER ELEVEN.........................**119**

BABY SHOWERS AND OTHER PRE-BABY CELEBRATIONS: IDEAS AND ETIQUETTE 119

CHAPTER TWELVE........................**128**

CHOOSING THE RIGHT HEALTH CARE PROVIDER FOR YOUR ANTENATAL CARE..................128

CHAPTER THIRTEEN **138**

PREPARING YOUR HOME FOR THE ARRIVAL OF YOUR NEWBORN 138

CHAPTER FOURTEEN....................**146**

BREASTFEEDING BASICS: GETTING OFF TO A GOOD START.................146

CHAPTER FIFTEEN **164**

MAINTAINING YOUR RELATIONSHIP WITH YOUR PARTNER AS NEW PARENTS 164

CHAPTER SIXTEEN.........................**173**

SLEEP SOLUTIONS FOR PREGNANT
WOMEN AND NEW MOMS 173

CHAPTER SEVENTEEN **182**

POSTPARTUM CARE: TAKING CARE
OF YOURSELF AFTER CHILDBIRTH 182

CHAPTER EIGHTEEN **192**

RETURNING TO WORK AFTER
MATERNITY LEAVE: BALANCING
CAREER AND MATERNITY.............192

CHAPTER NINETEEN.......................**202**

BUILD A SUPPORT NETWORK OF
OTHER FUTURE AND NEW PARENTS
....202

CHAPTER TWENTY 211

PARENTING PHILOSOPHIES AND
APPROACHES: FINDING WHAT
WORKS FOR YOU AND YOUR BABY
....211

Chapter One

THE STAGES OF PREGNANCY

Pregnancy is a remarkable journey that brings new life into the world. It is a complex process that takes place in several stages, from design to delivery. Each stage is characterized by distinct changes in the mother's body and the development of the growing fetus. In this article, we'll explore the stages of pregnancy, highlighting key milestones and the transformations that occur along the way.

1. Design and Implementation:

The pregnancy journey begins with conception, which occurs when a sperm cell fertilizes an egg cell. It usually happens during sex, where millions of sperm are released into the vagina. Only a few of them reach the fallopian tubes, where the egg waits to be fertilized. Once fertilization has taken place, the fertilized egg, now called a zygote, begins to divide rapidly as it travels down the fallopian tube towards the uterus. Around the fifth day after fertilization, the zygote implants into the lining of the uterus, beginning the next stage of pregnancy.

2. **FIRST QUARTER:**

The first trimester is a crucial period of development. During this stage, the major organ systems of the embryo begin to form. Cells divide and differentiate, creating the basis of the future body. At the end of the first month, the embryo has a beating heart and basic features such as the brain, spinal cord and limbs begin to take shape. The placenta, a vital organ that provides nutrients and oxygen to the fetus, also develops during this period. At the end of the third month, the embryo is called a fetus and all major organs and body structures are present.

3. **SECOND QUARTER**:

As the second trimester begins, the mother typically experiences a decrease in early pregnancy symptoms like nausea and fatigue. This trimester is often considered the most pleasant for expectant mothers. The fetus continues to grow rapidly, and its movements become more noticeable. During this stage, the mother's womb expands as the uterus expands to accommodate the growing fetus. Midway through pregnancy, the baby's gender can usually be determined by ultrasound. The fetus develops a layer of fine hair called lanugo and its skin becomes covered with a protective waxy substance called vernix.

4. **THIRD QUARTER**:

The third trimester brings the final stages of pregnancy, with the fetus rapidly gaining weight and preparing for life outside the womb. The mother's belly grows and she may experience increased discomfort due to the pressure on her internal organs. Fetal movements become more pronounced but may seem more restricted as space becomes limited. In preparation for birth, the fetus settles into a head-down position, preparing for the journey through the birth canal. Towards the end of the third trimester, Braxton Hicks contractions may occur, which are training contractions preparing the uterus for labor.

5. LABOR AND DELIVERY:

The culmination of the pregnancy journey is labor and delivery. The labor is divided into three stages: the early phase, the active phase, and the pushing phase. The early stage involves the cervix gradually thinning and dilating, preparing for childbirth. In the active stage, the contractions become stronger and more frequent, helping to push the baby through the birth canal. Finally, during the pushing phase, the mother exerts an effort to push the baby. Once the baby is born, the umbilical cord is cut and the placenta is expelled, marking the end of childbirth.

Chapter two

NAVIGATING COMMON PREGNANCY SYMPTOMS AND DISCOMFORTS

Pregnancy is a beautiful and transformative journey, but it can also come with its own set of discomforts and symptoms. As the body undergoes significant changes to support the growth and development of a new life, it is common for women to experience various physical and emotional challenges during pregnancy. Although every woman's experience is unique, there are several common symptoms that many pregnant women experience. Understanding and learning to manage these symptoms can help expectant mothers better manage their pregnancy and enjoy this special time.

Morning sickness is one of the most well-known symptoms of pregnancy.

Despite its name, morning sickness can occur at any time of the day. It usually presents as nausea and vomiting, especially during the first trimester. Although the exact cause is unknown, hormonal changes are thought to play an important role. To relieve morning sickness, it is advisable to eat small, frequent meals and avoid spicy or fatty foods. Ginger, whether in the form of tea, ginger ale, or ginger candy, can also provide relief. If morning sickness becomes severe and interferes with daily life, it is important to see a health care provider.

Fatigue is another common complaint during pregnancy, especially at the start and end. The body goes through tremendous physical and hormonal changes, which can lead to increased fatigue and a general feeling of lack of energy. To fight against fatigue, it is crucial for pregnant women to favor rest and sleep. Taking short naps during the day, delegating tasks, and asking for support from loved ones can help manage this symptom. Engaging in light physical activities, such as prenatal yoga or walking, can also boost energy levels.

As the pregnancy progresses, many women experience back pain and pelvic pain. The growing belly puts pressure on the back and pelvis, causing discomfort and sometimes even pain. Maintaining good posture, using supportive pillows while sleeping, and avoiding heavy lifting can help alleviate these symptoms. Engaging in gentle exercises that strengthen core and back muscles, with guidance from a medical professional, can also provide relief. Applying heat packs or receiving prenatal massages from trained professionals are additional options pregnant women can explore.

One of the most iconic signs of pregnancy is a growing belly, which can lead to stretch marks. These reddish or purplish streaks on the skin occur due to the stretching and expansion of the skin to accommodate the growing fetus. Although stretch marks are a natural part of pregnancy, keeping the skin hydrated with creams or oils can help reduce their severity. Staying hydrated and maintaining healthy weight gain during pregnancy can also contribute to overall skin health.

Another discomfort that many pregnant women experience is swelling in the feet and ankles, especially during the later stages of pregnancy. This swelling, called edema, occurs due to increased blood volume and pressure on the veins. To minimize swelling, it is recommended to elevate the feet as much as possible and to avoid standing or sitting for long periods of time. Wearing comfortable, supportive shoes and avoiding tight clothing can also help improve circulation. Drinking plenty of water and consuming foods low in sodium can prevent excessive water retention.

Pregnancy hormones can also affect the digestive system, leading to constipation and hemorrhoids. To relieve constipation, it's important to eat a high-fiber diet with plenty of fruits, vegetables, and whole grains. Staying hydrated and exercising regularly can also promote regular bowel movements. Hemorrhoids, which are swollen blood vessels in the rectal area, can be managed by avoiding prolonged sitting, incorporating more fiber into the diet, and using over-the-counter creams or ointments under the guidance of a healthcare professional.

Finally, the emotional well-being of pregnant women should not be overlooked. Pregnancy can cause a range of emotions, from excitement and joy to anxiety and mood swings. It is essential that pregnant women prioritize self-care.

Chapter three

THE EMOTIONAL ROLLER MOUNTAINS

Pregnancy is a beautiful journey filled with joy, anticipation and excitement. However, it is also a time of significant hormonal changes that can lead to mood swings and emotional ups and downs. It is essential that expectant mothers and their loved ones understand and manage these mood swings to ensure a healthy and happy pregnancy experience.

Mood swings during pregnancy are mainly caused by hormonal fluctuations. The increase in hormones, such as estrogen and progesterone, affects neurotransmitters in the brain, leading to changes in mood and emotions. Additionally, the physical and emotional stress of pregnancy, coupled with anxiety about impending motherhood responsibilities, can contribute to mood swings.

It is essential to remember that mood swings during pregnancy are normal and common. However, if mood swings become severe, prolonged, or interfere with day-to-day functioning, it is essential to seek professional help as they could be a sign of a more serious condition such as depression or anxiety.

To effectively manage mood swings during pregnancy, consider the following strategies:

1. Communication: Open and honest communication with your partner, family and friends can be extremely beneficial. Inform them of your emotional state and explain that it is the result of hormonal changes. Sharing your feelings can provide you with a support and understanding system, helping you feel more validated and less alone.

2. Self-Care: Prioritize self-care activities that help you relax and unwind. Engage in activities that bring you joy and peace, such as taking walks, reading a book, practicing prenatal yoga or meditation, or taking a warm bath. Taking care of your physical and emotional well-being is crucial during this time.

3. Healthy lifestyle: A well-balanced diet, regular physical activity and adequate sleep play an important role in stabilizing mood. Nutrient-dense

foods, such as fruits, vegetables, whole grains, and lean proteins, provide needed energy and promote emotional well-being. Exercise releases endorphins, the "feel-good" hormones, and helps reduce stress. Additionally, ensuring adequate sleep can improve mood and overall mental health.

4. Stress management: Pregnancy can lead to stress and anxiety, which can intensify mood swings. It is essential to identify stress triggers and develop

effective coping mechanisms. Techniques such as deep breathing exercises, mindfulness, journaling, and seeking social support can help manage stress levels and promote emotional stability.

5. Seek professional help: If your mood swings are severe, persistent, or accompanied by symptoms of depression or anxiety, it's crucial to see a medical professional. They can assess your condition, provide appropriate advice and suggest

treatments if needed. Remember that asking for help is a sign of strength and a proactive step in ensuring a healthy pregnancy.

6. Join support groups: Connecting with other pregnant women who are going through similar emotions can be very beneficial. Joining support groups or online communities can provide a safe space to share experiences, seek advice, and receive emotional support. It helps normalize your

feelings and reminds you that you are not alone on this journey.

7. Practice relaxation techniques: Incorporate relaxation techniques into your daily routine. Deep breathing exercises, progressive muscle relaxation, guided imagery, or prenatal massage can help alleviate stress, reduce anxiety, and promote emotional well-being.

8. Keep a Journal: Writing down your thoughts and feelings in a journal can serve as a therapeutic outlet. It allows you to express yourself freely and helps you gain clarity and understanding of your feelings. Plus, reflecting on your experiences throughout pregnancy can be a treasured memory for years to come.

Remember that pregnancy is a temporary phase and mood swings will eventually subside. However, being proactive in managing your emotional well-being can make travel more enjoyable and fulfilling. Surround yourself with a support network, prioritize self-care, and seek professional help when needed. By implementing these strategies, you can navigate the emotional roller coaster of pregnancy with greater ease and grace.

Another key aspect to consider is the role of the partner and loved ones in supporting an expectant mother through mood swings. Partners can play a crucial role by being understanding, patient and empathetic. It is important for partners to educate themselves about the hormonal changes and emotional challenges that come with pregnancy. By actively participating in the journey, partners can provide emotional support and help alleviate stress.

HOW PARTNERS CAN SUPPORT DURING PREGNANCY:

1. Educate yourself: Educate yourself about the physical and emotional changes that occur during pregnancy. Understand that mood swings are a normal part of the process and not a reflection of personal shortcomings. This knowledge will help you respond with empathy and compassion.

2. Be present and attentive: Be available for open, non-judgmental conversations. Create a safe space for your partner to express their feelings and concerns. Actively listen and

validate their emotions. Sometimes just being there to lend a listening ear can make a significant difference.

3. Show empathy and understanding: Put yourself in your partner's shoes and try to understand the intensity of the emotions she may be feeling. Avoid dismissing or minimizing her feelings. Instead, reassure her and let her know that you are there to support her unconditionally.

4. Helping with daily chores: Pregnancy can be physically exhausting, especially as the baby bump grows. Offer to help with household chores, cooking and shopping. By sharing responsibilities, you can alleviate some of the stress and allow your partner to focus on their well-being.

5. Go with her to appointments: Attend prenatal appointments with your partner. This demonstrates your involvement and interest in

pregnancy. It also keeps you updated on the progress of the pregnancy and any potential issues that may arise.

6. Take care of yourself together: Encourage and participate in self-care activities with your partner. Take a walk together, practice relaxation techniques or enjoy a prenatal yoga class. By engaging in these activities as a couple, you can strengthen your bond and promote emotional well-being.

7. Seek counseling together: Attend childbirth education classes or parenting workshops together. Learning more about the different stages of pregnancy, labor and team parenting can help you both feel more prepared and confident. It also allows you to share experiences and support each other along the journey.

8. Be patient and understanding: Remember that mood swings can be difficult for both the mother-to-be and the partner. Patience and understanding are essential.

Remember that these mood swings are temporary and a natural part of the process. Respond with love and support, even in difficult times.

By actively participating in your partner's emotional well-being and maintaining open communication, you can strengthen your relationship and create a supportive environment for her throughout pregnancy.

Chapter four

NUTRITIONAL TIPS FOR HEALTHY PREGNANCY AND FETAL DEVELOPMENT

Pregnancy is a critical time in a woman's life, and good nutrition plays a vital role in ensuring a healthy pregnancy and optimal fetal development. The expectant mother's diet should be well balanced and provide essential nutrients to support the growth and development of the baby. Here are some nutritional tips to support healthy pregnancy and fetal development.

1. Folic Acid: Adequate intake of folic acid is crucial early in pregnancy as it helps in the formation of the baby's neural tube, which later develops into the brain and spinal cord. Include folic acid-rich foods like leafy green vegetables, citrus fruits, legumes, and fortified cereals in your diet. It is also recommended to take a folic acid

supplement before and during the onset of pregnancy.

2. Iron: Iron is essential for the production of red blood cells, which carry oxygen to the baby. Pregnant women need greater amounts of iron to meet their increased blood volume. Include iron-rich foods like lean meats, poultry, fish, fortified cereals, beans, and spinach in your diet. To improve iron absorption, eat foods rich in vitamin C such as oranges, strawberries and tomatoes.

3. Calcium: Calcium is essential for the development of baby's bones and teeth. It also helps in maintaining the bone health of the mother. Include dairy products like milk, cheese, and yogurt in your diet. If you're lactose intolerant or follow a vegan diet, opt for calcium-fortified, plant-based dairy alternatives like almond or soy milk. Additionally, include calcium-rich foods like broccoli, kale, and tofu.

4. Protein: Protein is the building block of cells and tissues, and is vital for

baby's growth and development. Include good sources of protein in your diet, such as lean meats, poultry, fish, eggs, dairy products, legumes, nuts and seeds. Aim for a variety of protein sources to ensure you're getting a wide range of essential amino acids.

5. Omega-3 fatty acids: Omega-3 fatty acids, especially DHA (docosahexaenoic acid), are essential for baby's brain and eye development. Include fatty fish like salmon, sardines

and trout in your diet. If you are a vegetarian or don't eat fish, you can opt for vegetarian sources of omega-3 fatty acids like chia seeds, flax seeds and walnuts. Consult your health care provider before taking omega-3 supplements.

6. Hydration: Staying hydrated during pregnancy is crucial as it promotes the baby's development and helps prevent common pregnancy discomforts like constipation and urinary tract infections. Drink enough

water throughout the day and include hydrating foods like fruits and vegetables in your diet.

7. Fiber: Constipation is a common problem during pregnancy due to hormonal changes. Including fiber-rich foods like whole grains, fruits, vegetables, legumes, and nuts can help prevent constipation and promote regular bowel movements.

8. Avoid certain foods: Certain foods pose a health risk to the baby during pregnancy. Avoid raw or undercooked meats, seafood, and eggs, as they may contain harmful bacteria. Minimize consumption of fish high in mercury such as shark, swordfish, king mackerel and tilefish, as mercury can be harmful to the baby's developing nervous system. Limit your caffeine intake and completely avoid alcohol and smoking.

9. Prenatal Supplements: In addition to a healthy diet, your health care provider may recommend prenatal supplements to ensure you meet your nutritional needs. Prenatal vitamins usually contain essential nutrients like folic acid, iron, calcium, and other vitamins and minerals necessary for a healthy pregnancy.

10. Regular prenatal care: Finally, it is essential to attend regular prenatal checkups. with your healthcare provider. Prenatal care allows healthcare professionals to closely

monitor your health and your baby's development. They can provide personalized advice, address any concerns or complications, and make necessary adjustments to your diet and lifestyle.

During prenatal exams, your health care provider may perform various tests and screenings to ensure your well-being and that of your baby. They will monitor your weight gain, blood pressure, and check for any signs of gestational diabetes or preeclampsia. These visits also provide an opportunity to discuss your nutritional intake, address any discomfort or symptoms you may be experiencing, and receive advice on exercise and general prenatal wellness.

Remember to communicate openly with your healthcare provider about your diet, any food aversions or cravings, and any difficulties you may have in maintaining a healthy diet. They can provide valuable information and recommend appropriate dietary modifications or supplements based on your specific needs.

In addition to nutrition, prenatal care encompasses other essential aspects of a healthy pregnancy. This includes managing stress levels, getting enough rest, regular physical activity (with your health care provider's approval), and good hygiene to reduce the risk of infections.

Maintaining a healthy lifestyle and nutritious diet during pregnancy not only promotes your baby's growth and development, but also supports your overall well-being. It can help prevent complications such as premature birth, low birth weight, and developmental issues. It also lays the foundation for a healthy postpartum recovery.

It is important to remember that every pregnancy is unique and individual nutritional needs may vary. Consulting a registered dietitian specializing in prenatal nutrition can provide you with personalized advice tailored to your particular situation.

Chapter five

STAYING ACTIVE WHILE PREGNANT: SAFE EXERCISE AND FITNESS ROUTINES

Staying active during pregnancy is crucial for maintaining a healthy lifestyle and supporting the well-being of mother and baby. Regular exercise can help relieve common pregnancy discomforts, improve overall fitness, and prepare the body for labor and delivery. However, it is important to prioritize safety and choose appropriate exercises and fitness routines that are suitable for pregnant women. In this article, we will discuss safe exercises and fitness routines to stay active during pregnancy.

Before beginning any exercise program during pregnancy, it is essential to consult with a health care provider or obstetrician. They can provide personalized advice based on your specific medical history and any potential risks or complications. In general, if you were physically active before getting pregnant, you will probably be able to continue exercising during pregnancy, but modifications may be necessary.

1. Walking: Walking is a low impact exercise that can be easily incorporated into a daily routine. It helps improve cardiovascular fitness, maintain a healthy weight, and strengthen leg muscles. Aim for at least 30 minutes of brisk walking most

days of the week, but listen to your body and adjust the intensity and duration as needed.

2. Prenatal Yoga: Prenatal yoga focuses on gentle stretching, relaxation, and breathing techniques, which can help improve flexibility, reduce stress, and prepare the body for childbirth. Look for specialized prenatal yoga classes or videos led by certified instructors who have experience with pregnant women.

3. Swimming: Swimming and water aerobics are great choices for pregnant women because they provide a low-impact, full-body workout while supporting the weight of your growing belly. Water exercises help relieve swelling and joint pain and reduce the risk of overheating since water keeps the body cool.

4. Prenatal Pilates: Prenatal Pilates focuses on strength, flexibility, and body alignment. It can help improve posture, balance and stability during

pregnancy. Be sure to join a class specifically designed for pregnant women or work with a qualified instructor who can modify the exercises to suit your changing body.

5. Stationary Bike: Using a stationary bike is a safe way to get a cardiovascular workout without putting undue strain on your joints. Adjust the resistance and pace to your comfort level and avoid sitting in a position that puts pressure on your abdomen.

6. Strength training: Light to moderate strength training can be beneficial during pregnancy, but it is important to use proper form and avoid heavy weights which can strain joints or lead to injury. Focus on exercises that target major muscle groups, such as squats, lunges, modified push-ups, and bicep curls.

7. Kegel exercises: Kegel exercises strengthen the pelvic floor muscles, which can help prevent urinary incontinence and support the pelvic

organs during pregnancy and childbirth. To do Kegels, you simply squeeze and hold the muscles you would use to stop the flow of urine. Hold the position for a few seconds, then release. Repeat several times throughout the day.

Regardless of the exercise chosen, pregnant women should take certain precautions to ensure their safety:

- Stay hydrated and avoid overheating. Drink plenty of water before, during, and after exercise, and avoid exercising in hot, humid environments.

- Wear comfortable, supportive clothing and properly fitting shoes to reduce the risk of falls and injury.

- Warm up before exercising and cool down afterwards to avoid muscle strain.

- Avoid exercises that involve lying flat on your back after the first trimester, as this can put pressure on the vena cava, a major blood vessel that can affect blood flow to the baby.

- Listen to your body and modify or stop any exercise that causes pain, dizziness, shortness of breath, or twitching.

Chapter six

PREPARING FOR LABOR AND CHILDBIRTH

Preparing for Labor and Birth: What You Need to Know

Pregnancy is an incredible journey filled with anticipation, joy, and some nerves. As your due date approaches, it is essential to prepare yourself physically, emotionally and practically for the experience of labor and birth. While every woman's birth experience is unique, understanding what to expect and taking some steps can help you feel more confident and empowered during this transformative event. In this article, we'll walk you through some essential aspects of preparing for labor and childbirth.

1.Education and knowledge

One of the best ways to prepare for work is to educate yourself about the process. Attend childbirth education classes or workshops that provide comprehensive information about pregnancy, labor, and birth. These classes often cover various pain management techniques, breathing exercises, and labor positions. Additionally, they can offer information about medical procedures and cesarean delivery, allowing you to make informed decisions.

2.Make a birth plan

Creating a birth plan allows you to communicate your preferences and expectations to your healthcare provider and support team. Discuss your birth plan with your obstetrician or midwife, who can guide you in understanding your options and maternity policies. A birth plan typically includes your preferences for pain management, fetal monitoring, positions during labor, and any special requests you may have, such as delayed cord clamping or immediate skin-to-skin contact.

3.A physical training

Maintaining good physical health during pregnancy can contribute to a smoother labor. Get regular exercise appropriate for your stage of pregnancy, such as walking, prenatal yoga, or swimming. These activities can improve your endurance, flexibility, and overall well-being. Also, practice relaxation techniques and breathing exercises, which can help manage pain during labor and promote a calm state of mind.

4. Emotional support

Labor and birth can be emotionally intense experiences. Surround yourself with a strong support network, including your partner, family members and friends. Joining a prenatal support group or seeking advice from a doula can provide additional emotional support and comfort. Communicate openly with loved ones about your feelings and fears, allowing them to offer you the comfort and encouragement you may need.

5. Prepare your hospital bag

As your due date approaches, pack a hospital bag with the essentials for you and your baby. Include comfortable clothes, toiletries, nursing bras, and items to help you relax, such as music, a favorite pillow, or soothing scent. Don't forget to pack clothes and blankets for your newborn, as well as necessary documents, such as your ID and insurance information. Having everything ready in advance will ease the stress when it's time to get to the hospital.

6. Know the signs of labor

Familiarize yourself with the signs of labor, including regular contractions, rupture of membranes (water breaking), and bloody sight.

Understanding these indicators will help you distinguish between true labor and false labor, allowing you to make timely decisions about when to go to the hospital or birth center.

7.Contact your health care provider

Maintaining open communication with your healthcare provider is crucial during pregnancy, especially as your due date approaches. Attend regular prenatal appointments, ask questions, and discuss any concerns or unusual symptoms you may be experiencing. Be proactive in discussing your birthing preferences and understanding your healthcare provider's approach to labor and birth. Building a relationship of trust with your provider will improve your confidence and comfort during this critical time.

Remember that every birth experience is different and unexpected situations can arise. Flexibility and a positive mindset are key. By preparing yourself physically, emotionally, and practically, you can enter the process of labor and birth feeling empowered and ready to embrace this life-changing event.

Chapter seven

UNDERSTANDING PRENATAL SCREENINGS AND TESTS

Prenatal screenings and tests play a crucial role in ensuring the health and well-being of the expectant mother and the developing fetus. These medical procedures are designed to assess the risk of certain genetic conditions, birth defects, and other potential complications during pregnancy. By providing valuable information, prenatal screenings and tests enable healthcare professionals to provide appropriate care and support to expectant parents.

Prenatal screenings are usually done during the first and second trimesters of pregnancy. They aim to identify the likelihood of certain genetic disorders or chromosomal abnormalities in the fetus. One of the most common prenatal screenings is the first trimester screening, which combines a blood test and an ultrasound. During this screening, the mother's blood is analyzed to measure specific proteins and hormones. Additionally, an ultrasound is done to measure the thickness of the nuchal translucency, which is the fluid-filled space at the back of the baby's neck. By analyzing the results of these tests, healthcare professionals can estimate the risk of conditions such as Down syndrome and trisomy 18.

Another prenatal screening test is the quad screen, which is usually done between weeks 15 and 20 of pregnancy. This blood test measures levels of four substances in the mother's blood, including alpha-fetoprotein (AFP), human chorionic gonadotropin (HCG), estriol, and inhibin A. Abnormal levels of these substances may indicate the presence of certain birth defects or genetic conditions. disorders, such as neural tube defects and Down syndrome.

In addition to prenatal screenings, prenatal diagnostic tests are available for more definitive results. These tests are usually done if screening results indicate an increased risk of a genetic condition or birth defect. One of the best-known prenatal diagnostic tests is amniocentesis, which is usually performed between weeks 15 and 20 of pregnancy. During this procedure, a small amount of amniotic fluid is extracted using a needle under ultrasound guidance. The fluid contains fetal cells that can be tested for chromosomal abnormalities, genetic disorders, and neural tube defects. Although amniocentesis provides very accurate results, it carries a small risk of complications such as miscarriage.

Another common diagnostic test is chorionic villus sampling (CVS), which is usually performed between weeks 10 and 13 of pregnancy. CVS involves taking a sample of the placental tissue (chorionic villi) transcervically or transabdominally. Similar to amniocentesis, CVS allows the detection of chromosomal abnormalities and genetic disorders. It should be noted that CVS carries a slightly higher risk of miscarriage compared to amniocentesis.

It is important to understand that prenatal screenings and tests are optional and that the decision to undergo them is a personal choice for the future parents. The health care provider plays a crucial role in providing accurate information about the benefits, risks, and limitations of these procedures, allowing parents to make informed decisions based on their personal circumstances.

It is also essential to consider the ethical implications of prenatal screenings and tests. While these procedures offer valuable information about the health of the fetus, they can also present parents with difficult decisions about whether to continue or terminate a pregnancy. It is crucial that healthcare professionals provide non-directive advice and support to parents, ensuring that they have access to comprehensive information and guidance throughout the decision-making process.

Chapter eight

CREATE A BIRTH PLAN ADAPTED TO YOUR PREFERENCES AND NEEDS

Creating a birth plan is an essential step in preparing for the arrival of your baby. It allows you to communicate your preferences and needs to your healthcare team, ensuring that your birthing experience matches your wishes as closely as possible. By taking the time to develop a comprehensive birth plan, you can feel more empowered and in control on this transformative journey. Here are some key considerations to help you create a birth plan that matches your preferences and needs.

1. **inquire**:

Before creating a birth plan, it is crucial to gather information about the different birthing options available to you. Attend childbirth classes, read books, and check out reliable online resources to learn more about the different stages of labor, pain management techniques, and potential interventions. Understanding the possibilities will help you make informed decisions and adapt your birth plan accordingly.

2.**Choose your place of birth**:

Decide where you feel most comfortable giving birth. Options include a hospital, birth center, or home birth. Consider factors such as your medical history, the level of medical intervention you desire, and your comfort level with each setting. Make sure the location you choose supports the birth experience you envision.

3.pain management:

Think about how you plan to manage pain during labour. Options range from non-drug techniques such as breathing exercises, massage, and hydrotherapy to drug-based approaches such as epidurals or nitrous oxide. Consider your pain tolerance, personal preferences, and the potential benefits and risks associated with each method to make an informed decision.

4. Working environment:

Consider your ideal work environment and communicate your preferences. Would you like dim lights, soothing music or a specific aroma? Discuss these details with your healthcare provider and birthing facility to ensure they can accommodate your requests and create a calming atmosphere.

5. **Support people**:

Decide who you want by your side during labor and delivery. This may include your partner, a family member, or a doula. Clearly state their roles and responsibilities in your birth plan, as they will play a vital role in providing emotional and physical support throughout the process.

6.Delivery stations:

Research and explore various birthing positions that you find attractive. Discuss these options with your healthcare provider and include your preferences in the birth plan. Having the freedom to move and adopt positions that are comfortable for you can facilitate a smoother labor and delivery.

7.Interventions and Procedures:

Consider your position on routine interventions and procedures such as continuous fetal monitoring, episiotomy, or the use of forceps or vacuum extractors. Discuss the pros and cons of these interventions with your health care provider and outline your preferences in the birth plan.

8. Power Preferences:

Indicate your preferences for feeding your baby immediately after birth. Indicate whether you plan to breastfeed or bottle-feed and indicate your desire for skin-to-skin contact and delayed cord clamping. This information will help the healthcare team respond to your wishes and support your food choices.

9.**Unexpected scenarios**:

Recognize that the birth can sometimes deviate from the original plan. Discuss possible alternative scenarios with your health care provider and state your preferences in case interventions or procedures become necessary. Flexibility is key, and understanding your options ahead of time will help you make informed decisions in unforeseen situations.

ten. **Postpartum care**:

Consider your postpartum care preferences, including whether you prefer rooming with your baby, the type of aftercare you desire, and your position on circumcision, if any.

Communicate these preferences in your birth plan to ensure a smooth transition into the postpartum phase.

Remember that a birth plan serves as a guide, but it is important to remain flexible as circumstances may change during labour. Discuss your birth plan with your health care provider well in advance to make sure they know your preferences and can provide any advice or information you need. By preparing a complete birth plan that aligns.

Chapter nine

DEALING WITH PREGNANCY-RELATED COMPLICATIONS AND HIGH-RISK SITUATIONS

Pregnancy is a miraculous and transformative journey in a woman's life. However, it can also lead to unexpected challenges and complications. Dealing with pregnancy-related complications and high-risk situations requires careful management, support and a proactive approach to ensure the well-being of mother and baby. In this article, we'll explore some strategies for dealing with these challenges.

Above all, it is crucial for women to establish a strong support system made up of healthcare professionals, family and friends. Regular prenatal care is essential to monitor the progress of the pregnancy and identify any potential complications early on.

It is essential to find an experienced obstetrician or midwife who specializes in high-risk pregnancies and can provide the necessary medical advice and interventions.

Open and honest communication with the health care provider is paramount. It is important to ask questions, voice concerns and actively participate in the decision-making process. Understanding the potential risks and complications associated with pregnancy enables women to make informed choices and actively engage in their own care. Establishing a relationship of trust with the care provider ensures that the woman's needs and preferences are accommodated throughout the pregnancy.

Learning about the specific complication or high-risk situation is empowering. The more a woman knows about her condition, the better equipped she is to manage it. Trusted sources such as reputable medical websites, books, and support groups can provide valuable information and emotional support. However, it is important to consult health professionals for personalized advice and recommendations.

Taking care of physical and emotional well-being is crucial during high-risk pregnancies. This includes eating a healthy, balanced diet, practicing proper exercise, and getting enough rest. You may need to make certain changes to your lifestyle, such as avoiding certain foods or activities that may pose a risk to pregnancy. Rest and relaxation techniques like prenatal yoga, meditation, or deep breathing exercises can help reduce stress and promote overall well-being.

Seeking emotional support is equally important. Pregnancy can be an emotionally difficult time, especially when faced with complications or high-risk situations. Joining support groups or seeking advice can provide a safe space to share experiences, fears and emotions. Connecting with other women who are going through similar circumstances can be extremely comforting and reassuring.

Preparing for the possibility of premature labor or prolonged bed rest is crucial for women facing high-risk pregnancies. Creating a support network that can help with childcare, household chores, and transportation can alleviate some of the stress and ensure that needed rest is obtained. Planning ahead, packing a hospital bag, and discussing birth plans with the healthcare provider can help reduce anxiety and prepare for any potential scenarios.

It is essential to stay alert and be aware of the warning signs that may indicate a potential problem. Regularly monitoring fetal movements, noting any symptoms or abnormal changes, and reporting them promptly to the health care provider can make a significant difference in effectively managing complications. Trusting your instincts and seeing a doctor whenever there is a problem is vital.

Finally, maintaining a positive mindset and focusing on the joys and excitement of pregnancy can help overcome the challenges. Engaging in activities that bring joy and relaxation, such as prenatal massages, gentle walks in nature, or the pursuit of hobbies, can provide a much-needed emotional boost. Cultivating a positive support network and sharing the joys and triumphs of the pregnancy journey can also contribute to a more optimistic outlook.

Chapter ten

ROLE OF PARTNERS

The role of a partner during pregnancy and childbirth is crucial and encompasses emotional, physical and practical support. Pregnancy and childbirth are transformative experiences for both mother and partner, and being actively involved in the process can strengthen their bond and contribute to a positive birth experience. In this article, we will explore the different aspects of the partner's role throughout the journey of pregnancy and childbirth.

Emotional support is one of a partner's main responsibilities during this time. Pregnancy is often accompanied by a range of emotions, including joy, anxiety, and sometimes even fear. The partner can be a pillar of strength, offering comfort, understanding and a listening ear. They can attend prenatal appointments, actively engage in conversations about the baby's development, and provide a safe space for the mother to express her feelings and concerns.

During pregnancy, a partner can be actively involved in preparing for the baby's arrival. This includes attending childbirth education classes together, learning about the different stages of labor and discussing birth preferences. By being knowledgeable about the process, the partner can ease any fears or anxieties and provide guidance and support during labor.

Physical support is another essential role played by the partner. Pregnancy can bring discomfort and physical challenges, especially during the later stages. Partners can help by offering back massages, foot massages, or helping with household chores. They can also encourage the mother to maintain a healthy lifestyle by exercising regularly and eating nutritious meals.

As the due date approaches, the role of the partner becomes more important during labor and delivery. They can help the mother time contractions, pack needed items for the hospital or birthing center, and ensure a calm, relaxing environment. Partners can also act as advocates for the mother's birth plan, communicating her preferences to the medical team and providing support during medical interventions if needed.

During labour, the presence of the partner can have a profound impact on the mother's experience. Holding hands, offering words of encouragement, and ensuring constant presence can help create a sense of security and reduce anxiety. Partners can help with breathing exercises, position changes, and offer comforting measures such as ice cubes or a cool washcloth. Their unwavering support and reassurance can contribute to a more positive birthing experience.

In the event of medical interventions or complications, partners can play a crucial role in decision-making. They can help gather information, ask questions, and provide support as the couple navigates unexpected circumstances. The presence and active involvement of the partner can bring a sense of calm and confidence in difficult times.

After childbirth, the partner's role continues in supporting the mother in her recovery and adjustment to her new role as parent. This may involve helping with newborn care, assisting with breastfeeding, or providing emotional support during postpartum mood swings. Partners can also take on household responsibilities, allowing the mother to rest and bond with the baby.

Chapter eleven

BABY SHOWERS AND OTHER PRE-BABY CELEBRATIONS: IDEAS AND ETIQUETTE

Baby showers and other baby showers have become an integral part of welcoming new life into the world. These joyous occasions bring friends and family together to celebrate the impending arrival of a baby and shower expectant parents with love, support and gifts. If you're planning a baby shower or other baby shower, here are some ideas and etiquette tips to make it a memorable and enjoyable event.

1. Choose the right theme: Selecting a theme can add an element of fun and cohesion to the celebration. Take into account the preferences of the future parents, the gender of the baby (if known) or a neutral theme. Popular themes include "Welcome to the

Jungle", "Twinkle, Twinkle Little Star" or "Oh, Baby!" You can incorporate the theme into invitations, decorations, games, and even the cake.

2. Invitations: Send out invitations well in advance to ensure guests can save the date. Include all necessary details, such as date, time, location, topic (if applicable), and any specific instructions or requests. You can also include registry information if the parents created one. Consider digital

invitations to save on paper and make RSVPs easier.

3. Venue and decorations: Baby showers can be held at a variety of locations, such as the home of the expectant parents, a parent's house, a restaurant, or a rented venue. Decorate the space according to the chosen theme or with a color scheme that reflects the baby's gender or a neutral palette. Balloons, banners, centerpieces and tablecloths can create a festive atmosphere.

4. Food and drink: Plan a menu that meets the tastes and dietary restrictions of the guests. Bites, appetizers and bite-sized treats are popular choices for baby showers. Include a mix of sweet and savory options, and don't forget to have a cake or cupcakes for the centerpiece. Offer a variety of non-alcoholic beverages, such as mocktails, infused water, or sparkling fruit juices.

5. Games and Activities: Baby shower games are a great way to entertain

guests and create a happy atmosphere. Classic games like "Guess the baby food", "Baby Bingo" or "Baby Name Scramble" are always a hit. You can also set up a craft station where guests can decorate onesies or create personalized baby mobiles. Consider the preferences and physical limitations of expectant parents when choosing games or activities.

6. Give gifts: The main purpose of a baby shower is to celebrate the imminent arrival of the baby and to

support expectant parents by providing essential items for their new journey. Create a registry to help guests choose appropriate gifts, or suggest a theme for gifts, such as books, clothing, or baby items. Encourage guests to bring practical and useful gifts for the baby's first year. Don't forget to express your gratitude and send thank you notes to all attendees after the event.

7. Etiquette Considerations: When hosting a baby shower or baby

shower, it is important to consider the wishes and circumstances of the expectant parents. Check to see if they have any preferences regarding the guest list, freebies, or general tone of the event. Be aware of any cultural or religious traditions that may influence the celebration. Avoid surprises that could cause unnecessary stress or discomfort for future parents.

8. Inclusive celebrations: It is essential to create an inclusive environment

where all guests feel welcome and comfortable. Consider attendees' diverse backgrounds and preferences when planning the event. Respect different dietary restrictions, provide accessible accommodations where necessary, and avoid games or activities that may exclude or embarrass some people. Celebrate the joy of a new life while being aware of each other's needs and sensitivities.

Chapter twelve

CHOOSING THE RIGHT HEALTH CARE PROVIDER FOR YOUR ANTENATAL CARE

Choosing the right health care provider for your prenatal care is one of the most important decisions you will make on your pregnancy journey. Prenatal care plays a vital role in ensuring the health and well-being of mother and baby. This involves regular check-ups, screenings and counseling to promote healthy pregnancy and childbirth. To make an informed decision, there are several factors to consider when selecting a healthcare provider.

First, you will need to choose between an Obstetrician-Gynecologist (OB-GYN) or a Registered Nurse Midwife (CNM). Both professionals are qualified to provide prenatal care, but they have different approaches. OB-

GYNs are doctors who specialize in women's reproductive health and pregnancy. They can manage high-risk pregnancies, perform surgeries if needed, and have access to advanced medical interventions. On the other hand, CNMs are registered nurses with specialized training in prenatal care and childbirth. They focus on providing personalized and holistic care and often emphasize natural childbirth options.

Consider your own preferences and priorities when deciding between an OB-GYN and a CNM. If you have a pre-existing medical condition or are planning a high-risk pregnancy, an OB-GYN might be the most appropriate choice due to their medical expertise. However, if you want a more natural and personalized approach to your pregnancy, a CNM may be the right solution.

Once you have decided on the type of health care provider, you can start searching for specific individuals or practices. Ask for recommendations from friends, family, or other trusted sources who have had positive experiences with prenatal care. Online ratings and reviews can also provide insight into patient experiences. Look for vendors who have a good reputation, excellent communication skills, and a caring attitude.

Accessibility and convenience are crucial factors to consider. Prenatal care involves regular checkups throughout pregnancy, so you'll want to choose a provider whose office is easily accessible and not too far from your home. Consider the availability of meeting times that fit your schedule. Also, check to see if the provider has a reliable system for emergency situations or after-hours care.

It is important to assess the level of experience and expertise of the health care provider. Find out about their qualifications, years of experience in prenatal care, and their approach to handling various situations. Ask if they have experience dealing with specific complications or conditions related to your pregnancy. A competent and experienced provider can reassure you and advise you throughout your pregnancy journey.

Consider the type of facility or practice where the provider operates. Do they work in a hospital, birthing center or private clinic? Each setting has its own advantages and considerations. Hospitals provide access to a wide range of medical resources and specialists, which can be beneficial in the event of complications. Birth centers often offer a more home-like environment with an emphasis on natural childbirth. Private clinics can provide a more personalized experience and shorter wait times for appointments.

Compatibility between you and your healthcare provider is crucial for a positive prenatal care experience. Schedule an initial consultation or interview with potential providers to assess their communication style, approach to care, and ability to address your concerns. You should feel comfortable asking questions and expressing your preferences. Mutual trust and respect are essential for a successful doctor-patient relationship.

Finally, consider the financial aspect of prenatal care. Contact your insurance provider to determine which health care providers and services are covered by your plan. Find out about any disbursements, co-payments or deductibles you may be responsible for. Choosing a provider that is part of your insurance network can help reduce costs and streamline the billing process.

Chapter thirteen

PREPARING YOUR HOME FOR THE ARRIVAL OF YOUR NEWBORN

Preparing your home for the arrival of your new baby is an exciting and important task. As you eagerly anticipate your little one's arrival, it's essential to create a safe, comfortable and nurturing environment for them. From baby safety to organizing the essentials, there are several steps you can take to ensure your home is ready for your newborn. Here are some tips to help you prepare your home for the newest addition to your family.

First and foremost, safety should be your top priority. Start by securing your baby home. Start by securing all electrical outlets with safety covers to prevent your curious little one from inserting their fingers or objects into them. Install baby gates at the top and bottom of stairs to prevent falls. Make sure heavy furniture is anchored to the walls to prevent tipping. Consider installing window guards to prevent accidents, especially if you live in an upper level apartment. Remove any small objects or choking hazards from the floor and ensure that all cabinets and drawers are secured with childproof locks.

Next, creating a cozy and comfortable nursery for your newborn is essential. Choose a room that is well ventilated and receives natural light. Paint the walls with non-toxic, baby-safe paint and opt for soft, soothing colors that promote a calm and relaxing environment. Choose functional furniture, such as a crib, changing table and comfortable rocking chair to feed and soothe your baby. Invest in a quality mattress that provides adequate support and firmness. Arrange the furniture in a way that allows easy access to all the essentials.

Organizing baby essentials is another crucial step in preparing your home.

Stock up on necessary items such as diapers, wipes, baby clothes, bibs and blankets. Create designated storage areas for each item to ensure easy access when needed. Label baskets or drawers for specific purposes to keep everything organized. Consider setting up a diaper changing station in a convenient place, with diapers, wipes, diaper rash cream, and a changing pad.

As your baby grows, you will find that he accumulates a significant number of toys and accessories. To keep these items organized, incorporate storage solutions such as bins, shelves, and toy boxes into the nursery and other areas of your home. Dedicate specific spaces for toys, books, and clothes to maintain order and reduce clutter. Regularly review your baby's things and donate or store outgrown items to keep your home tidy and organized.

In addition to safety and organization, creating a nurturing environment for your newborn is crucial. Consider adding soft lighting options such as nightlights or dimmers to create a soothing ambiance during late night feedings and diaper changes. Hang curtains or blinds that allow for light control and privacy. Play soft, soothing music in the nursery to promote relaxation and promote sleep. Make sure the temperature in the nursery is comfortable and suitable for your baby. Keep a comfy chair or armchair in the bedroom for nighttime feedings and comforting your little one.

Finally, take care of yourself and establish a support system. Preparing your home for a newborn can be physically and emotionally demanding. Ask for help from your partner, family members or close friends to prepare the nursery and complete the necessary tasks. Accept help when offered and prioritize self-care to ensure you are well rested and ready to care for your baby.

Chapter fourteen

BREASTFEEDING BASICS: GETTING OFF TO A GOOD START

Breastfeeding is a natural and beautiful way to feed your baby. It provides many benefits to both mother and baby, including essential nutrients, bonding, and a stronger immune system. However, getting off to a good start with breastfeeding can sometimes be difficult for new mothers. In this article, we'll explore the basics of breastfeeding to help you establish a successful and enjoyable breastfeeding journey.

1. Educate yourself: Before your baby arrives, take the time to educate yourself about breastfeeding. Attend breastfeeding classes or workshops, read reliable books or online resources, and talk to experienced mothers. Understanding the benefits, techniques and common challenges of

breastfeeding will help you feel more confident and prepared.

2. Seek support: Having a support system in place is crucial during the early stages of breastfeeding. Contact your partner, family members or friends who can encourage you and help you concretely. Also, consider contacting a lactation consultant or joining a breastfeeding support group. These professionals can provide personalized advice and address any concerns or difficulties you may encounter.

3. Skin-to-skin contact: Immediately after birth, try to establish skin-to-skin contact with your baby. This practice promotes bonding and triggers your baby's natural instinct to seek out the breast. Keep your baby on your chest, preferably with minimal clothing between you, allowing warmth and direct access to the breast. Skin-to-skin contact also helps regulate your baby's body temperature and stabilize their heart rate and breathing.

4. Early initiation: Breastfeeding should ideally be initiated within the first hour after birth. Babies are often alert during this time and have a strong instinct to latch on. Take advantage of this period to offer your breast to your baby. It may take a few tries before your baby latches on properly, but don't be discouraged. Seek help from a healthcare professional or lactation consultant to ensure proper latching and positioning.

5. Establish a good latch: A good latch is essential for successful breastfeeding. When latching on, your baby's mouth should cover not only the nipple, but also a significant portion of the areola. This ensures that your baby gets enough milk and reduces the risk of nipple pain or damage. If you are having difficulty latching on, seek advice from a lactation consultant who can provide practical assistance.

6. Demand feeding: Newborns have small stomachs and need to feed frequently. It is important to feed your baby on demand, that is, to feed him whenever he shows signs of hunger. Watch for signs such as rooting, sucking motions, or putting hands to mouth. On-demand feeding helps establish your milk supply and ensures that your baby receives adequate nutrition.

7. Monitor diaper production: A good indicator of your baby's feeding

success is his diaper production. During the first few days, your baby should have at least one wet diaper per day of life (eg, one wet diaper on the first day, two wet diapers on the second day). By day five, your baby should have at least six wet diapers and several stools. If you are concerned about your baby's diaper bulk, consult a healthcare professional.

8. Take care of yourself: Breastfeeding requires energy and hydration. Make

sure you eat a balanced diet, drink plenty of fluids, and get enough rest. Consider setting up a comfortable nursing station with water, snacks, and items you may need during breastfeeding sessions, such as breast pads, nipple cream, or a pillow breastfeeding. Remember that taking care of yourself is key to maintaining healthy milk supply.

Remember that breastfeeding is a learning process for you and your baby. It may take time and practice to establish a comfortable and effective breastfeeding routine. Do not hesitate to ask for help or seek advice whenever you need it. With the right support, patience, and perseverance, you can overcome any initial challenges and enjoy a successful breastfeeding journey. Here are some additional tips to help you through the process:

9. Pay attention to breastfeeding positions: Try different breastfeeding positions to find the most comfortable

for you and your baby. Some popular positions include the cradle hold, football hold, side-lying position, and relaxed breastfeeding. The right position can make a significant difference in your comfort level and your baby's ability to latch on effectively.

10. Treat Breastfeeding Discomfort: Although breastfeeding shouldn't be painful, some mothers may experience temporary discomfort or pain in the first few days. If you

experience pain while breastfeeding, it is important to identify and treat the underlying cause. This could be due to a poor latch, engorgement, or even a potential infection such as mastitis. Consult a lactation consultant or healthcare professional to help resolve any discomfort and ensure a positive breastfeeding experience.

11. Recognize hunger cues: Understanding your baby's hunger cues can help you meet her food needs quickly. Early signals of hunger

include increased alertness, rooting, licking lips, or bringing hands to mouth. Crying is a late hunger signal, so try to start nursing before your baby becomes too hungry and restless.

12. Pumping and storing breast milk: If you need to be away from your baby or want to build up a supply of stored milk, pumping can be a useful tool. Invest in a good quality breast pump and learn how to use it effectively. Follow good hygiene practices when

expressing and storing breast milk to ensure its safety for your baby. Label and date containers of milk and store them in the refrigerator or freezer according to directions.

13. Be patient with milk supply: It is common for new mothers to worry about their milk supply. Remember that breast milk production works on the basis of supply and demand. The more you breastfeed or pump, the more milk your body will produce. Avoid supplementing with formula or

using pacifiers in the first few weeks as this can interfere with establishing a strong milk supply. Instead, focus on frequent and effective breastfeeding sessions to boost milk supply.

14. Take note of growth spurts: Babies go through growth spurts where they may seem hungrier and want to breastfeed more frequently. These periods can be difficult and can cause you to doubt your milk supply. Rest assured that growth spurts are normal and temporary. They allow your baby

to increase your milk supply to meet his growing needs. Offer the breast whenever your baby shows signs of hunger during these times.

15. Weaning: At some point you may decide to begin the weaning process. Whether you choose to wean gradually or abruptly, it is essential to do so in a way that is comfortable for you and your baby. Gradual weaning allows your milk supply to decrease gradually, reducing the risk of engorgement or mastitis. Seek help

from a lactation consultant or your healthcare provider if you need advice on how to wean effectively.

Remember that every breastfeeding journey is unique and it is essential to trust your instincts and do what is right for you and your baby. Celebrate your accomplishments along the way, whether it's successfully latching on, increasing your milk supply, or simply enjoying the special bond breastfeeding brings. Breastfeeding is a gift you give to yourself and your baby, providing nourishment, comfort and love. Embrace the journey, seek support when needed, and cherish the beautiful moments shared during this precious time.

Chapter fifteen

MAINTAINING YOUR RELATIONSHIP WITH YOUR PARTNER AS NEW PARENTS

Nurturing your relationship with your partner as new parents

Becoming parents is an incredible journey filled with joy, love and new challenges. Amid the excitement and demands of caring for a newborn, it's essential to remember to nurture your relationship with your partner. The arrival of a baby can bring significant changes to your relationship dynamics, but with effort and communication, you can strengthen your bond and navigate this new chapter together. In this article, we'll explore some essential tips for nurturing your relationship with your partner as new parents.

1. Prioritize communication: Effective communication is the foundation of a healthy relationship, especially during

this time of transformation. Make it a priority to communicate openly and honestly with your partner. Share your feelings, concerns and needs. Also actively listen to your partner's thoughts and feelings. Clear and compassionate communication will promote understanding and avoid misunderstandings.

2. Show your appreciation: Being new parents comes with a lot of responsibilities and sleepless nights. In the midst of these challenges, it is

essential to appreciate everyone's efforts. Acknowledge and express gratitude for your partner's contribution to parenting and running the household. A simple "thank you" or kind gesture can go a long way in strengthening your bond.

3. Make time for each other: Balancing parenting and personal time can be tricky, but setting aside quality time for both of you is essential. Schedule regular dates or evenings at home where you can focus on

reconnecting and enjoying each other's company. This dedicated time allows you to nurture your romantic relationship and strengthens your identity as a couple beyond being parents.

4. Share responsibilities: Parenting is a team effort, and sharing responsibilities is crucial for both partners to feel supported and valued. Discuss and divide tasks such as feeding, diaper changes and bedtime routines. Sharing the workload not

only eases everyone's burden, but also strengthens your bond as you work together toward a common goal.

5. Take care of yourself: Taking care of yourself individually is essential to maintaining a healthy relationship. As new parents, it's easy to get caught up in your child's needs and neglect self-care. However, remember that by prioritizing your well-being, you will be better equipped to nurture your relationship. Find time for the activities you enjoy, seek support from

family and friends, and make sure you get enough rest and relaxation.

6. Keep the Romance Alive: Even though your focus is on your child, remember to keep the romance alive in your relationship. Surprise yourself with small gestures of love and affection. Set aside intimate times to reconnect physically and emotionally. By nurturing the romantic aspect of your relationship, you will maintain a strong bond that can withstand the challenges of parenthood.

7. Seek support: It is essential to recognize that you don't have to do this alone. Seek support from family, friends or parent support groups. Sharing experiences and challenges with others can provide valuable insight and reassurance. Consider seeing or attending couples therapy if you are having significant relationship issues. Professional advice can help you overcome any difficulties and strengthen your bond.

8. Be patient and forgiving: The transition to parenthood is a learning process for both partners. It's normal to make mistakes and experience frustrations along the way. Practice patience and forgiveness, both for yourself and for each other. Remember that you are a team and working together through the ups and downs will bring you closer in the long run.

Chapter sixteen

SLEEP SOLUTIONS FOR PREGNANT WOMEN AND NEW MOMS

Sleep Solutions for Pregnant Women and New Moms

Pregnancy and the first stages of motherhood are joyful and transformative experiences for women. However, they are often accompanied by a myriad of physical and emotional changes that can disrupt sleep patterns. Sleep is crucial for the well-being of mother and baby, and finding effective sleep solutions becomes a priority. In this article, we'll explore various strategies and tips to help pregnant women and new moms get the rest they need.

During pregnancy, hormonal fluctuations, physical discomfort and frequent trips to the bathroom can make it difficult to get a good night's sleep. As pregnancy progresses, finding a comfortable sleeping position can become increasingly difficult. However, there are several strategies that can alleviate these issues and promote better sleep.

First, investing in a comfortable and supportive mattress and pillows is essential. Pregnancy pillows, such as full pillows or wedge pillows, can provide extra belly support and help relieve back pain. Experimenting with different pillow arrangements can help pregnant women find a comfortable position that reduces discomfort and promotes better sleep.

Creating a relaxing bedtime routine can also contribute to better sleep. Taking a warm bath, practicing gentle stretches, or engaging in a calming activity like reading or listening to soothing music can help signal the body that it's time to relax. It is advisable to avoid stimulating activities, such as using electronic devices or watching television, before bed, as the blue light emitted by screens can interfere with the sleep-inducing hormone melatonin.

Maintaining a healthy sleeping environment is equally important. Keeping the bedroom cool, dark, and quiet can promote better sleep. Using blackout curtains, earplugs, or a white noise machine can help create a more conducive sleeping environment. Additionally, wearing loose, breathable sleepwear and using comfortable bedding can improve comfort levels.

As the baby arrives, sleep patterns are further disrupted. Frequent newborn feeding, diaper changes and irregular sleep schedules can make new moms feel exhausted. However, there are strategies that can help new moms get through this difficult phase and maximize their rest.

An effective approach is to prioritize sleep and rest whenever possible. This means accepting the help of partners, family members or friends to share the responsibilities of caring for the baby. Shifting tasks and seeking support can free up valuable time for mothers to catch up on sleep or take short naps during the day.

Establishing a consistent sleep routine for baby and mom can also be beneficial. Babies thrive on predictability, and having a structured sleep schedule can help regulate their sleep patterns over time. Coordinating the mother's sleep routine with that of the baby can increase the likelihood of getting longer periods of uninterrupted sleep.

Creating an environment conducive to sleep is crucial for mother and baby. Making sure the bedroom is dark, quiet, and at a comfortable temperature can facilitate better sleep. Using blackout curtains, white noise machines, or soothing lullabies can help create a soothing ambiance that promotes relaxation and sleep.

For breastfeeding mothers, finding a comfortable position for nighttime feedings can make a significant difference in sleep quality. Using nursing pillows or experimenting with different breastfeeding positions can help reduce physical fatigue and discomfort during nighttime feedings, making it easier for mother and baby to get back to sleep.

Chapter seventeen

POSTPARTUM CARE: TAKING CARE OF YOURSELF AFTER CHILDBIRTH

After the exhilarating and transformative experience of childbirth, it is crucial for new mothers to prioritize postpartum care and focus on their own physical and emotional well-being. The postpartum period, often referred to as the fourth trimester, can be challenging as the body adjusts to hormonal changes, heals after childbirth, and adjusts to the demands of caring for a newborn. By taking proactive steps to care for themselves, women can promote recovery, regain strength, and enjoy a positive postpartum experience.

One of the most important aspects of postpartum care is rest. Pregnancy and childbirth are physically and emotionally demanding, and the body needs time to heal. New mothers should strive to get enough sleep and take frequent naps whenever possible. Accepting help from family members and friends can be invaluable during this time, allowing mothers to have dedicated rest periods.

Feeding the body with a healthy and balanced diet is another essential part of postpartum care. Providing the nutrients needed to support healing and lactation is crucial. Including foods high in iron, calcium, protein, and vitamins can help replenish depleted stores. Staying hydrated is also vital, especially for breastfeeding mothers, as breastfeeding can increase fluid needs. Prioritizing self-care often means making sure nutritious meals and snacks are readily available.

Exercise and gentle movement can aid in postpartum recovery. Engaging in activities such as walking, yoga, or postpartum-specific exercise programs can help strengthen the body, improve circulation, and improve mood. However, it is important to consult a medical professional before beginning any exercise routine to ensure that it is safe for individual circumstances.

Emotional well-being plays an important role in postpartum care. Postpartum hormonal changes, combined with the demands of caring for a newborn, can lead to a range of emotions, including baby blues or postpartum depression. It is crucial that new mothers prioritize self-care activities that promote mental and emotional health. This may include seeking support from loved ones or joining new parent support groups, engaging in relaxation techniques such as deep breathing or meditation, and finding time for activities that bring joy and relaxation.

Another essential aspect of postpartum care is physical healing. Proper wound care for caesarean section or episiotomy incisions, if required, is essential to prevent infection and promote healing. Good hygiene practices, including regular showers and frequent changing of sanitary napkins, are important during the postpartum period. It is essential to watch for any unusual symptoms or signs of complications and seek prompt medical attention to ensure a healthy recovery.

Breast care is especially important for breastfeeding mothers. Ensuring a good latch, using nipple creams or ointments to relieve pain, and maintaining good breast hygiene are key parts of postpartum care. Seeking help from lactation consultants or support groups can help with breastfeeding challenges and promote a successful nursing relationship.

In addition to physical care, new mothers should prioritize compassion and self-acceptance during the postpartum period. It's important to remember that every woman's postpartum journey is unique and it's normal to experience a range of emotions and physical changes. Comparing yourself to others or striving to have unrealistic expectations can be detrimental to overall well-being and the recovery process. Practicing self-compassion and seeking out positive affirmations can promote a healthy self-image and build confidence during this time of transformation.

In conclusion, postpartum care is essential for new mothers to prioritize their physical and emotional well-being after childbirth. By focusing on rest, nutrition, exercise, emotional support, wound care, breastfeeding support, and self-compassion, women can aid recovery, regain strength, and enjoy the joys of motherhood. Seeking advice from healthcare professionals and creating a support network can further improve the postpartum experience. Remember, talk.

Chapter eighteen

RETURNING TO WORK AFTER MATERNITY LEAVE: BALANCING CAREER AND MATERNITY

Returning to work after maternity leave can be both an exciting and challenging time for new mothers. Balancing career and motherhood requires careful planning, support, and a willingness to adapt to new routines and responsibilities. It's a journey that many women embark on, and while it may seem daunting at first, with the right mindset and strategies in place, it's possible to thrive both personally and professionally. .

One of the first steps to successfully balancing career and motherhood is to plan ahead. Before returning to work, it is essential to fully understand your priorities and goals, both at home and in your professional life.

Take the time to assess what is most important to you and your family, and how you can align your career aspirations with your new role as a mother. This may involve reassessing your career path, considering flexible work arrangements, or exploring new opportunities that are better suited to your current lifestyle.

Communication is key during this time of transition. It's crucial to have open and honest conversations with your employer about your expectations and needs as a working mother. Discussing flexible work hours, remote work options, or reduced hours can help create a supportive and accommodating work environment. Many companies now recognize the importance of retaining experienced employees and are willing to work with mothers to find a balance that works for everyone.

Building a support network is essential for working mothers. Reach out to other working mothers in your organization or community. Sharing experiences, tips and strategies can be invaluable in overcoming the challenges of balancing work and motherhood. Additionally, consider seeking out professional support services such as childcare providers, family members, or trusted friends who can help with childcare responsibilities when needed. . Having reliable and trustworthy caregivers will give you peace of mind while you focus on your career.

Another important aspect of balancing career and motherhood is self-care. As a new mother, it's easy to prioritize your child's needs and your work, neglecting your own well-being. However, taking care of yourself is essential to maintaining a good work-life balance. Set aside time for activities that recharge you, whether it's exercising, practicing mindfulness, or pursuing hobbies you enjoy. Remember that a happy and fulfilled mother is better equipped to handle the demands of her career and her family.

Effective time management is crucial for working mothers. Develop strategies to prioritize tasks, set realistic goals, and delegate when necessary. Effective time management skills can help reduce stress and allow you to make the most of the limited time you have. Use tools like calendars, to-do lists, and productivity apps to stay organized and focused.

Flexibility and adaptability are essential qualities to cultivate as an active mother. Recognize that there will be times when unexpected challenges arise or when the demands of work and family seem overwhelming. Be prepared to adjust your plans and expectations as needed, and be kind to yourself when things don't go your way. Remember that you are doing your best and that it is okay to ask for help or ask for help when needed.

Finally, don't forget to celebrate successes, big and small. Balancing career and motherhood is no small feat, and it's important to recognize and celebrate your accomplishments along the way. Whether it's a successful project at work or a milestone your child has reached, take the time to savor these moments and reflect on how far you've come.

Returning to work after maternity leave can be a difficult transition, but with careful planning, open communication, a strong support network and a commitment to self-care, it is possible to find balance and flourish in her career and motherhood. Remember that every mother's journey is unique and finding what works best for you and your family is key. By prioritizing your needs, setting realistic expectations, and accepting the joys and challenges that come with life.

Chapter nineteen

BUILD A SUPPORT NETWORK OF OTHER FUTURE AND NEW PARENTS

Building a support network of other future and new parents is essential to navigating the joys and challenges of parenthood. It provides a sense of community, emotional support, and valuable resources that can make the journey smoother and more fulfilling.

From sharing experiences and advice to finding comfort in knowing you're not alone, a support network can be a lifeline during this transformative phase of life.

The transition to parenthood can be overwhelming, especially for new parents. The physical, emotional and logistical demands can leave individuals feeling isolated and insecure. However, by actively seeking out and maintaining connections with other future and new parents, one can create a strong support network that will help them navigate the ups and downs of this incredible journey.

One of the most effective ways to build a support network is to join local parent groups or attend prenatal classes. These places make it possible to meet other parents who are going through similar experiences. Through shared discussions and activities, bonds can be formed and a sense of camaraderie can develop. These groups often continue to meet even after childbirth, allowing parents to have ongoing support as their children grow.

Social media platforms also provide a way to connect with other parents. There are many online communities dedicated to parenting where individuals can find advice, share stories and ask questions. Participating in these communities can help create virtual connections that can be just as valuable as face-to-face interactions. However, it is important to approach online interactions with caution, ensuring that the platforms are trustworthy and that the information shared is reliable.

Another beneficial step in building a support network is reaching out to friends and family who have recently become parents or are also expecting. These people can provide a familiar and reliable support network. They may have valuable insights and advice to share based on their own experiences, and their presence can provide a sense of comfort and reassurance during difficult times.

In addition to seeking support from others, it is equally important to offer support in return. Building a support network is a two-way street, and by actively engaging and being there for others, relationships within the network become stronger and more meaningful. By sharing your own experiences, offering help, and lending an empathetic ear, you can create a supportive environment where everyone benefits.

Scheduling regular meetings, both in person and online, is essential to maintaining and strengthening the support network. These gatherings can take the form of play dates, coffee get-togethers or simply informal get-togethers where parents can share their joys, concerns and challenges. Such interactions provide parents with the opportunity to learn from each other, celebrate milestones together, and encourage each other through difficult times.

Beyond emotional support, a network of other parents can also provide practical assistance. This could include sharing recommendations for local services such as pediatricians, daycare centers or baby stores. This may involve carpooling or swapping game dates to give yourself a break. With a support network, parents can rely on each other for advice, recommendations and help with day-to-day tasks, making the journey of parenthood more manageable.

Chapter twenty

PARENTING PHILOSOPHIES AND APPROACHES: FINDING WHAT WORKS FOR YOU AND YOUR BABY

Being a parent is a journey filled with joy, challenges and countless decisions. From the moment a baby is born, parents are faced with the task of nurturing and guiding their little one through the stages of life.

However, there is no one-size-fits-all approach to parenting. Each child is unique and each parent has their own beliefs and values. This is where parenting philosophies and approaches come into play.

Parenting philosophies are frameworks that help parents understand their role and guide their interactions with their child. They provide guidance and help parents make informed choices about how to raise their children. There are many parenting philosophies and approaches, each with its own set of principles and techniques.

A popular philosophy is attachment parenting. It emphasizes creating a strong emotional bond between parent and child through practices such as on-demand breastfeeding, co-sleeping and babywearing. Proponents of attachment parenting believe that meeting a baby's needs quickly and consistently promotes secure attachment and promotes emotional well-being.

On the other hand, some parents may follow a more structured approach, such as the Babywise method. This method emphasizes establishing a routine for eating, sleeping and playtime. It encourages parents to set boundaries and teaches babies to self-soothe and develop independent sleeping habits. Proponents of the Babywise method argue that it promotes a sense of security and predictability for both baby and parent.

Another philosophy is positive parenting, which aims to foster a respectful and loving relationship between parent and child. This involves setting clear boundaries, using positive reinforcement, and practicing open communication. Positive parenting aims to teach children valuable skills and values for life, such as empathy, self-discipline and problem solving.

Some parents may take a more holistic approach, such as mindful parenting. Mindful parenting emphasizes being fully present and engaged in the moment with your child. It encourages parents to listen to their own emotions and reactions and to respond to their child with compassion and understanding. Mindful parenting practices include meditation, self-reflection, and non-judgmental mindfulness practice.

It is important to note that no philosophy or approach is superior to the others. The most important thing is to find what works for you and your baby. Every child is different and every parent has their own strengths, limitations and cultural background. What works for one family may not work for another. Therefore, it's crucial to consider your child's temperament, your own values, and your unique family dynamics when choosing a parenting philosophy.

It should also be mentioned that parenthood is a dynamic process that evolves over time. What works for your baby in the first few months may not work as he gets older. It is essential to remain flexible and adaptable, being open to adjusting your approach as your child's needs change.

Ultimately, the key to successful parenting is creating a loving and nurturing environment where your child can thrive. This involves meeting their needs, providing guidance and support, and cultivating a strong, trusting relationship. By exploring different philosophies and approaches, you can gain insights and tools to help you navigate the difficult but rewarding journey of parenthood. Remember that there is no "right" way to parent, but by finding what works for you and your baby, you can create a beautiful bond that will last a lifetime.

Made in the USA
Columbia, SC
05 October 2023

23989434R00122